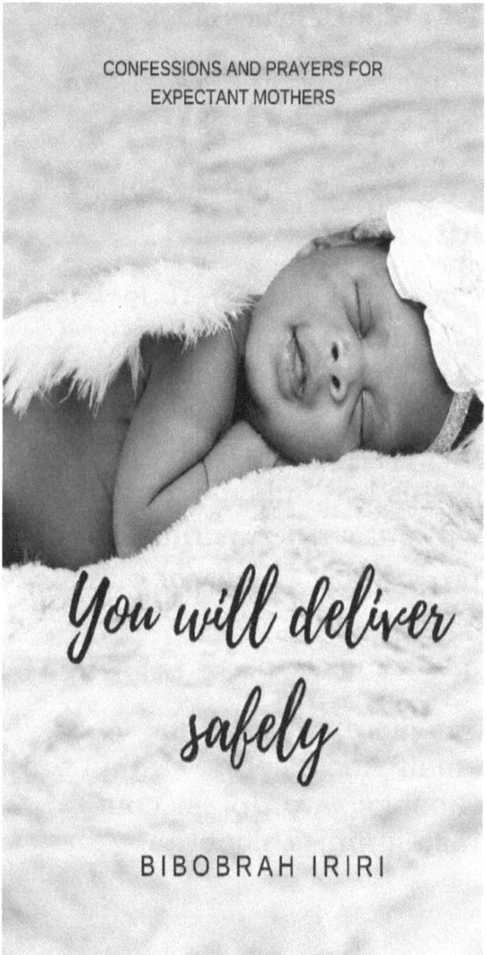

CONFESSIONS AND PRAYERS FOR
EXPECTANT MOTHERS

You will deliver safely

BIBOBRAH IRIRI

You Will Deliver Safely

Confessions and Prayers for Expectant Mothers

For more information
email: booksbybibo@gmail.com
Biboblogs.wordpress.com
Instagram: @bibobrah

CONTENTS

Introduction

For God has not given us a spirit of fear, but of power and of love and of a sound mind. 2 Timothy 1.7 NJKV

God's heart for you is good. He is a good gift giver. It is not God's plan for you to have a miscarriage or lose your child. I know because He has said in His word that none shall be barren or cast their young (Exodus 23.26). That includes you. If you had a miscarriage or traumatic birthing experience in the past, know this, God makes everything work out for your good. God is so good. His heart towards you is good. God is not responsible for your pain but if you would give it to Him, He will turn it into something beautiful.

The inspiration for this book came as what I can best describe as a quiet whisper 'you will deliver safely'. I did not hear an audible voice, but I knew in my spirit what I had heard.

Jesus is so amazing. He has so many promises for you and He wants you to get the right tools in your hands to win this victory. You don't have to have a bad experience when bringing

your children to the world.
Your previous experiences do
not define what will happen in
future.

If you will be 'crazy' enough to
believe, you will receive. *Is it
really that simple?* Follow me
on this journey and you will
have your miracle in your
hands in Jesus name.

CHAPTER ONE

The Father's Heart

[6] "For God
so [greatly] loved *and* dearly
prized the world, that
He [even] gave His [One and]
only begotten Son, so that
whoever believes *and* trusts
in Him [as Savior] shall not
perish, but have eternal life.
John 3.16 AMP

In May 2019, I had a dream. It was unlike any dream I had ever had before. I saw Jesus Christ, my Lord and Saviour. I know when we hear stories like this we want to ask about the fine details. *Do the pictures do*

Him justice? What does He look like? None of those thoughts crossed my mind.

The light from His presence was so radiant and no one told me, I knew instantly in whose presence I was. The light was so blinding that I could not stand. I could only see His feet as I lay flat on the floor. The light filled the entire room. He came closer and closer to me. As He came closer, I started to become aware of myself, aware of how frail and human I was. The thoughts grew louder and the fear palpable. I struggled to suppress the negative thoughts in my mind. For a spilt second, it felt as if I could not see the light anymore.

Instead of walking away, Jesus came closer and closer until He could put His hand in mine, and He did just that. Instantly I was lifted. He gave me strength to stand in His presence. He spoke to me and His words are the reason you are reading this book today. *'I want you to write to let people know how much I love them'.*

God wants you to know He's smitten, and it is all because of you. He conceived you in His heart before you were conceived in your mother's womb. He's so interested in every area of your life. He wants to be your Father and friend, lover and saviour. He wants to be all things to you.

In His presence, there is pure undiluted love. In my dream, I had a moment where I felt so inadequate but one touch from God and love radiated right through me. He loves me recklessly, as if I am the only person in this world. The good news is that He feels the same way about every single person on the planet and that includes you my friend.

God wants you to know in everything that He loves you. He knows you intimately. He

does not care about your past
because He has a good future
for you. He wants you to enjoy
your life here and most
importantly, Jesus wants to
spend eternity with you.

Jesus wants you to have a
wonderful birthing experience.
But what He is really after is
your heart and your life. In Him
is power to transform. You are
not too old or too young. You
are not too busy or idle. Not
worthless or forgotten, He
wants to give you a new name.

There's no greater love than the
love of Jesus Christ and He
wants you to know that love
(John 15.13)

It's so simple to be a part of
this beautiful family. As many
as believe He has given them
the power to become sons of
God (John 1.12). Please say
this prayer with me:

**Father I believe Jesus. I
believe that you died for me
and that you love me. I lay
down my life to you, all my
mistakes, my highs and lows.
I give my heart to you, come
into my heart. Come and be
the Lord of my life.**

Congratulations and welcome
home. I am so honoured to
welcome you into this family.

Jesus loves you. The idea of
love is embodied in the person
of Jesus. He created love; He is
love. I'm sure you are
wondering what a book about
pregnancy and childbirth has
to do with the love of God. I felt
it so important to start with
God's heart for you. His heart
for you is filled with good. He
loves you more than words can
describe.

When you were in sin, when
you did not know him, he took
a chance with you. He walked
to the cross, endured the
shame, and physical pain. The
gospel is simple. God so loved
the world that He gave his son,

that whoever believes in Him
would have everlasting life.

***You saw me before I was
born.
Every day of my life was
recorded in your book.
Every moment was laid out
before a single day had
passed. Psalm 139.16 NLT***

God's plans for you date back
to before you were born. Before
you were formed in your
mother's womb, He set you
apart for greatness. I pray that
as you read the pages of this
book, your mind is set free and
you embrace the love of God
whilst living above your fears.

CHAPTER TWO

Dealing with Fear

So far, we have established that God's will for you is good and that He is in love with you.

Fear in pregnancy may appear valid. Maybe you or someone you know had a bad experience, a miscarriage, stillbirth or perhaps the death of a young child. None of these are pleasant experiences. There might even be a deep-seated fear that you can't trace concerning pregnancy and delivery. Either way, God's word is light and when light

shines in the darkness,
everywhere is illuminated.

**We demolish arguments and
every pretension that sets
itself up against the
knowledge of God, and we
take captive every thought to
make it obedient to Christ. 2
Corinthians 10.5 NIV**

Fear many times starts as a
thought. A small niggling voice
in your head. You might not be
able to express it in words but
it's there, eating at the fabric of
your reality. It may even
present past experiences to
validate your fear. A previous
loss makes you more at risk a
second time. The baby (or

babies) in your womb grows and it feels like the fear is growing too. What a lie!

Thank God for a saviour who is so mindful of you. He has given you the victory and shown you how to war. God has protected your baby and you. Fear is not of God. In His perfect love, all fear dissipates (1John 4.18).

I am confident, that those who trust in God won't be put to shame. I am confident that if you put the word of God to work, you will see it work in your life.

God is no respecter of persons. What He has done for one, He will do for all. The devil might have lied to you, but this time is different. This time you shall know the truth and it will set you and your entire family free.

Speak out.

When those thoughts come, be sure to speak out. You may not feel like it. In fact, opening your mouth might be the last thing you want to do but open it anyway.

What do you speak? The word of God. *But Bibo, what if I don't know any verse?* Thankfully you have this book and I would highlight some promises that you can pray and profess over

your life and that of your
baby(babies).

CHAPTER THREE

The Potency of the Word

For the word of God *is* living and powerful, and sharper than any two-edged sword, piercing even to the division of soul and spirit, and of joints and marrow, and is a discerner of the thoughts and intents of the heart. Hebrews 4.12 NKJV

Can I tell you an open secret? The word of God is Jesus Himself. Stay with me, I will show you from scripture. When you speak the word of God, you call Jesus into the heart of every situation. That's why the devil would stop at nothing to make sure you don't get the word into your spirit and out of your mouth. The moment you can internalise His word and proclaim it, you release the same potency as if it were coming out of the mouth of God.

That is why Paul says in the scripture you just read that the word of God is alive. Jesus is alive. The word in your mouth can go deep, deep into the crevices of your broken heart.

What an amazing God we serve! He did not hide a single thing from us. The same power He

has, He gave to us (John
15.15).

**Now I saw heaven opened,
and behold, a white horse.
And He who sat on
him *was* called Faithful and
True, and in righteousness
He judges and makes war. His
eyes *were* like a flame of fire,
and on His head *were* many
crowns. He a name written
that no one knew except
Himself. He *was* clothed with
a robe dipped in blood, and
His name is called The Word
of God. And the armies in
heaven, clothed in fine linen,
white and clean, followed
Him on white**

horses. Now out of His mouth goes a sharp sword, that with it He should strike the nations. Revelations 19.11-15NKJV

Wow! Look at that vivid description of our loving savour. Our mighty man of war, *Yeshua hamashiach,* Jesus the anointed one. The Lion of the tribe of Judah. We can sit with this piece of scripture for days and still not be able to do it justice.

This time however, I want you to read a name that Jesus has- The word of God. Remember the open secret? Jesus is the word of God.

When He opens His mouth, the word of God oozes out. The sharp sword Paul likened the word of God to in Hebrews is the same one that comes out of the mouth of Jesus when He speaks. It is the same one that will come out of you as you pray and confess the word of God over yourself and your generation.

The word of God is alive. This means that every time you speak out the word, it goes to the root of the problem and like a surgeon's scalpel, dissects it, exposing things that ought not to be there.

It can uproot every seed and root of fear. God's plan for you is to have your children and to be sound physically and mentally to take care of them. How do I know? From Genesis to Revelation, the bible is filled with promises of divine protection and fruitfulness.

When God created man and woman, He commanded them to be fruitful and spoke a blessing over them that is still speaking today. Many things change but not our God. He is the same yesterday, today and forever. (Hebrews 13.8).

As you speak the word, it might feel like nothing has changed.

The fears may appear louder
and stronger but fix your eyes
on His promises. Things are
shifting even when you cannot
see it.

You might have wonderful
plans for your children, but
God's plan and purpose for
them is more beautiful than
words can fully articulate. God
will preserve you in
childbearing regardless of any
past experiences.

**Nevertheless, she will be
saved in childbearing if they
continue in faith, love, and
holiness, with self-control.1
Timothy 2.15 NKJV**

How to Use this Book

Please don't just scheme through the pages of this book. This book will require you to be bold and make confessions. I trust that as you trust in God, He will heal your heart and you will see His will made flesh in your life.

CHAPTER FOUR

God is your midwife

God shows us an image in Revelations 12 of things to come. But it also shows a nature and character of our God, that He is a midwife.

In this chapter of scripture, we see a woman crouched in pain with each wave of labour contractions. The pain was unbearable, but that was only a part of the problem. At her feet was the enemy, ready and waiting to kill her child.

Thank God that is not how the story ends. God takes the child Himself and keeps the woman

safe in a place He prepared for
her.

This is the nature of God. The
devil's plans and schemes will
all come to nothing because
Jesus is waiting to catch your
baby and keep you safe in
body, soul and spirit.

CHAPTER FIVE

The Blood Speaks

One night I went to bed tired. I had a regular day-eat, work, and now sleep. But something different happened that night. I was sleeping but it I kept tossing and turning. I felt like I was listening to a message, waking up and then going back to it. The Blood still speaks.

It felt as if the message was being downloaded into my spirit, awkward description, I know.

God was showing me that His blood still speaks and that His

people had become silent.
He reminded me of the
Passover in Exodus.
How the Children of Israel put
the blood of a lamb without
blemish on their door posts
and the angel of death passed
over them.

Scriptures say 'when I see the
blood I will pass over'
He reminded me that seeing in
the spirit is voice activated.
The blood on their door posts
raised a sound.
It defended them. It spoke out
that they were untouchable
and undeniably God's own.

It wasn't just a blob of red

blood on their doors.
It wasn't just visual.
The blood spoke!

He then went on to remind me
that He is the lamb of God who
takes away the sins of the
world. The explanation was so
detailed. I had never heard
anything like it.
He brought to my memory the
first murder. The Cain and Abel
story and how Abel's blood
spoke out to God almighty and
He heard.

If Abel, a man after the flesh,
could have his blood speak out,
how much more the blood of
Jesus?

So, speak out in victory!
Speak out in glorious
affirmation of the goodness of
God! Seal your borders with
your words!
Command your open heavens!

**Now the blood shall be a sign
for you on the houses where
you are. And when I see the
blood, I will pass over you;
and the plague shall not be
on you to destroy you when I
strike the land of Egypt.
Exodus 12:13 NKJV**

**Jesus the Mediator of the
new covenant, and to the
blood of sprinkling that
speaks better
things than *that of* Abel.
Hebrews 12.24 NKJV**

By faith he kept the Passover
and the sprinkling of blood,
lest he who destroyed the
firstborn should touch them.
Hebrews 11:28 NKJV

And He said, "What have you
done? The voice of your
brother's blood cries out to
Me from the ground.
Genesis 4:10 NKJV

For My flesh is food indeed,
and My blood is drink indeed.
He who eats My flesh and
drinks My blood abides in Me,
and I in him. John 6.55-56
NKJV

CHAPTER SIX

Confessions

We have seen that Jesus is the word of God. That He has so graciously given us the same power and authority to release His word on our behalf. With that understanding, we are going to speak into the universe, speak to our spirits, speak to our fears and deliver our miracle.

Every confession is linked to at least one anchor scripture. Sit with it, say it out loud, read it and pray with it. As the Lord lives and as you release God's word into your situation, you will have the fruit of your lips.

*"For as the rain comes down,
and the snow from heaven,
And do not return there,
But water the earth,
And make it bring forth and
bud,
That it may give seed to the
sower
And bread to the eater,
So shall My word be that
goes forth from My mouth;
It shall not return to
Me void,
But it shall accomplish what
I please,
And it shall prosper in the
thing for which I sent it.
Isaiah 55.10-11 NKJV*

1.Before my baby (babies) was
formed in my womb, God knew

him or her intimately. That means before I planned this pregnancy, God knew my children. I declare that my children are formed according to God's original plan. Every trimester of pregnancy progresses according to God's original design. Every cell, organ and system in my baby responds to the word of God. My child is whole in Jesus name. **Before I formed you in the womb I knew you, before you were born I set you apart; I appointed you as a prophet to the nations." Jeremiah 1.5 NKJV**

2. God is my child's(children's) midwife. He is there in the delivery room with me, ready to catch my baby (babies) in His loving arms. Therefore, we are safe in the arms of God. Nobody can snatch us from His loving embrace. **By You I have been upheld from birth; You are He who took me out of my mother's womb. My praise shall be continually of You. Psalm 71.6 NKJV**

3. God has assured me that no weapon formed against me shall prosper. He has given me authority to condemn whatever evil is lurking in my life. I stand

with authority today and speak over my life and that of my children, it is well. I will deliver safely. **No weapon formed against you shall prosper, And every tongue which rises against you in judgment You shall condemn. This is the heritage of the servants of the LORD, And their righteousness is from Me," Says the LORD. Isaiah 54.17 NKJV**

4.God's voice makes me give birth. The same voice that called the universe into existence has spoken over my birth and delivery. Therefore, everything concerning pregnancy and delivery is smooth and settled. I silence every contrary voice.

**Who is he who speaks and it comes to pass,
When the Lord has not commanded it?
Lamentations 3.37 NKJV**

**The voice of the LORD makes the deer give birth,
And strips the forests bare;
And in His temple everyone says, "Glory!" Psalm 29.9 NKJV**

4.There's no enchantment or spell against me or my baby (babies). No negative word or

counsel shall stand. Only God's word shall stand in my generation. I speak to all the generations in my loins, you shall hear the word of the Lord. You do not respond to any contrary voice. **For there is no sorcery against Jacob, Nor any divination against Israel.
It now must be said of Jacob And of Israel, 'Oh, what God has done!' Numbers 23.23**

5.God has sworn to fight my battles. I am victorious. God will contend against all who contend against me and He will save my children.

But thus says the LORD:

**"Even the captives of the
mighty shall be taken away,
And the prey of the terrible
be delivered;
For I will contend with him
who contends with you,
And I will save your children
Isaiah 49.25 NKJV.**

6.Children are a heritage from
God. My Children belong to
God. They will fulfil destiny
from their first cry. God gives
good gifts. *Can anyone tamper
with God's gifts or his heritage?*
The answer is no! Nothing
tampers with these gifts in my

womb. **Behold, children are a heritage from the LORD, The fruit of the womb is a reward. Psalms 127.3 NKJV**

Every good gift and every perfect gift is from above, and comes down from the Father of lights, with whom there is no variation or shadow of turning James 1.17NKJV

7. I am God's own. The apple of his eyes. Oh, how the Father loves me. I will not have another miscarriage/stillbirth. Affliction will not rise again the second time. **What do you conspire against the LORD?**

**He will make an utter end of it.
Affliction will not rise up a second time. Nahum 1.9 NKJV**

8. I am the redeemed of the Lord, bought with a price. This is the heritage of my family. I won't die in childbirth. I won't have complications. God will supervise my birthing experience Himself. I do not miscarry. I deliver at term.

No one shall suffer miscarriage or be barren in your land; I will fulfill the number of your days. Exodus 23.26 NKJV

9.God has not given me the spirt of fear. I have a sound mind concerning pregnancy, delivery and motherhood. God keeps my mind and fills it with love. I don't struggle with feelings of depression, anxiety or psychosis. God sheds His love in my heart to love my child(children). God's child(children). My mental health flourishes and blossoms as I have wisdom to take care of myself and be taken care of. **There is no fear in love; but perfect love casts out fear, because fear involves torment. But he who fears has not been made perfect in love. 1 John 4.18NKJV**

10.I will live and not die. It is that simple, my mouth will declare the works of God. I will teach my children about Jesus and His wondrous deeds. I will not die, I will live. My children will not die but live. **I shall not die, but live, and declare the works of
the LORD.Psalm118.17 KJV**

11. God is my strength. He gives me strength every single day of my pregnancy. His joy gives me strength. I radiate the glory of God. My baby(babies) feels this joy and leap(s) in my womb.

Then he said to them, "Go your way, eat the fat, drink

the sweet, and send portions to those for whom nothing is prepared; for this day is holy to our Lord. Do not sorrow, for the joy of the LORD is your strength."Nehemiah 8.10 NKJV

12. My pelvic muscles stretch to accommodate the weight of my baby. When labour comes, my body and mind is ready. I recover speedily from caesarean section. Neither me nor my baby has any complications. My body cooperates with the word of God. I will deliver safely! **And the midwives said to Pharaoh, "Because the Hebrew women *are* not like**

the Egyptian women; for
they *are* lively and give birth
before the midwives come to
them." Exodus 1.19 NKJV

Conclusion

Congratulations! Can you tell I am excited? Through the pages of this book, we have seen God's heart for you and your children. I am so excited because I know you will testify.

If you said the salvation prayer or want to share your testimonies, please email me booksbybibo@gmail.com. I would love to hear from you. Jesus loves you.

You won't lose another baby.

You won't bleed out.

You won't go home empty handed.

You will deliver safely.

You will have your babies and all who surround you will rejoice.

This book is for you if you've ever struggled with fear about your pregnancy or delivery.

It will end in praise!